94 Muscle Cramp Reducing Meal and Juice Recipes:

Stop Muscle Cramps Fast by Eating Vitamin Specific Foods

By

Joe Correa CSN

COPYRIGHT

This publication is designed to provide accurate and authoritative information in regard to the subject matter covered. It is sold with the understanding that neither the author nor the publisher is engaged in rendering medical advice. If medical advice or assistance is needed, consult with a doctor. This book is considered a guide and should not be used in any way detrimental to your health. Consult with a physician before starting this nutritional plan to make sure it's right for you.

ACKNOWLEDGEMENTS

This book is dedicated to my friends and family that have had mild or serious illnesses so that you may find a solution and make the necessary changes in your life.

94 Muscle Cramp Reducing Meal and Juice Recipes:

Stop Muscle Cramps Fast by Eating Vitamin Specific Foods

By

Joe Correa CSN

CONTENTS

ABOUT THE AUTHOR

After years of Research, I honestly believe in the positive effects that proper nutrition can have over the body and mind. My knowledge and experience has helped me live healthier throughout the years and which I have shared with family and friends. The more you know about eating and drinking healthier, the sooner you will want to change your life and eating habits.

Nutrition is a key part in the process of being healthy and living longer so get started today. The first step is the most important and the most significant.

INTRODUCTION

94 Muscle Cramp Reducing Meal and Juice Recipes: Stop Muscle Cramps Fast by Eating Vitamin Specific Foods

By Joe Correa CSN

The involuntary and rather painful condition of a contracted muscle that doesn't relax is something we have all experienced at least once in our life. Usually, the condition is quite harmless and it only lasts for a couple of minutes during which the person is unable to use the affected muscle.

Muscle cramps are often caused by difficult exercises, hard physical labor, dehydration, or use of certain medications. They can occur in almost every muscle in the body, especially in the leg and feet muscles. As I said earlier, most of the time muscle cramps are harmless, however, sometimes they can be related to some more serious medical condition like:

- Inadequate blood supply due to narrowed arteries causes muscle cramps during exercise.
- Nerve compression in the spine is related to muscle cramps while walking,

- Lack of minerals like potassium, calcium, or magnesium in your body can also lead to muscle cramps.

In some cases, it is highly recommended to visit a doctor, especially if you feel severe pain, muscle weakness, leg swelling, rashes or any other skin changes. Also, if you suffer from frequent muscle cramps that don't improve over time, medical attention is necessary.

Although muscle cramps can happen to everyone for various reasons, there are some risk factors that increase this painful condition. These factors include age, different medical conditions, and dehydration. Older people who lose their muscle mass are frequently affected by muscle cramps, even during some relatively easy physical activities. Pregnant women and people suffering from diabetes, thyroid or liver disorders also experience frequent and harmless muscle cramps. Finally, dehydration during long physical activities (especially in hot weather) is often the cause of muscle cramps.

There are a couple of simple steps that will help prevent muscle cramps. As mentioned above, muscle cramps are often related to dehydration which means that keeping your body fully hydrated all the time is crucial to avoid this painful condition. Drinking plenty of fresh juices will have an amazing effect on your entire body, including muscle cramps.

This collection of muscle cramp reducing juice recipes will keep your body hydrated all the time and provide a rich amount of different nutrients you need on a daily basis.

Take a couple of minutes every day to prepare one of these delicious recipes and forget about having muscle cramps once and for all.

COMMITMENT

In order to improve my condition, I *(your name)*, commit to eating more of these foods on a daily basis and to exercise at least 30 minutes daily:

- Berries (especially blueberries), peaches, cherries, apples, apricots, oranges, lemon juice, grapefruit, tangerines, mandarins, pears, etc.
- Broccoli, spinach, collard greens, sweet potatoes, avocado, artichoke, baby corn, carrots, celery, cauliflower, onions, etc.
- Whole grains, steel-cut oats, oatmeal, quinoa, barley, etc.
- Black beans, red bean beans, garbanzo beans, lentils, etc.
- Nuts and seeds including: walnuts, cashews, flaxseeds, sesame seeds, etc.
- Fish
- 8 – 10 glasses of water

Sign here

X_____

94 MUSCLE CRAMP REDUCING MEAL AND JUICE RECIPES

JUICES

1.   Watermelon Banana Juice

Ingredients:

1 cup of watermelon, diced

1 large banana, chunked

1 medium-sized wedge of honeydew melon

1 small ginger knob, peeled and chopped

1 medium-sized carrot, sliced

Preparation:

Cut the top of the watermelon. Cut lengthwise in half and then cut one large wedge. Peel it and cut into small cubes. Remove the seeds and fill the measuring cup. Wrap the rest in a plastic foil and refrigerate for later.

Peel the banana and cut into chunks. Set aside.

Cut the honeydew melon in half. Cut one large wedge and peel the peel it. Cut into small pieces and set aside. Wrap the rest of the melon in a plastic foil and refrigerate.

Peel the ginger and cut into small pieces. Set aside.

Wash and peel the carrot. Cut into thin slices and set aside.

Now, combine watermelon, banana, honeydew melon, ginger, and carrot in a juicer. Process until juiced.

Transfer to a serving glass and add some crushed ice before serving.

Enjoy!

Nutrition information per serving: Kcal: 230, Protein: 4.3g, Carbs: 75.8g, Fats: 1.2g

2.   Cucumber Pomegranate Juice

Ingredients:

1 large orange, peeled

1 large cucumber, sliced

1 cup of pomegranate seeds

1 cup of purple cabbage, torn

1 cup of sweet potatoes, cubed

4 oz of water

Preparation:

Wash the cucumber and cut into thick slices. Set aside.

Cut the top of the pomegranate fruit using a sharp knife. Slice down to each of the white membranes inside of the fruit. Pop the seeds into a measuring cup and set aside.

Peel the orange and divide into wedges. Set aside.

Wash the cabbage thoroughly under cold running water. Drain and torn with hands. Set aside.

Peel the sweet potato and cut into cubes. Fill the measuring cup and reserve the rest for another juice. Set aside.

Now, combine orange, pomegranate seeds, purple cabbage, sweet potatoes, and cucumber in a juicer and process until juiced.

Transfer to serving glasses and stir in the water. Add some ice cubes and serve immediately.

Enjoy!

Nutritional information per serving: Kcal: 251, Protein: 6.8g, Carbs: 73.1g, Fats: 1.5g

3.   Squash Raspberry Juice

Ingredients:

1 cup butternut squash, chopped

1 cup raspberries

2 cups cantaloupe, chopped

1 large apricot, chopped

1 large kiwi, peeled

Preparation:

Peel the butternut squash and cut in half. Scoop out the seeds using a spoon. Cut into small chunks and set aside. Reserve the rest for another juice.

Rinse the raspberries under cold running water using a large colander. Set aside.

Cut the cantaloupe in half. Scoop out the seeds and flesh. Cut two wedges and peel them. Chop into chunks and set aside. Reserve the rest of the cantaloupe in a refrigerator.

Wash the apricot and cut in half. Remove the pit and cut into chunks. Set aside.

Peel the kiwi and cut lengthwise in half. Set aside.

Now, combine squash, raspberries, cantaloupe, apricots, and kiwi in a juicer.

Transfer to serving glasses and add some ice before serving.

Enjoy!

Nutritional information per serving: Kcal: 193, Protein: 6.6g, Carbs: 59.1g, Fats: 2.3g

4.   Banana Apple Juice

Ingredients:

1 large banana, sliced

1 small Golden Delicious apple, cored

2 cups blueberries

1 large cucumber, sliced

3 oz water

Preparation:

Peel the banana and cut into small chunks. Set aside.

Wash the apple and remove the core. Cut into bite-sized pieces and set aside.

Place the blueberries in a colander and wash under cold running water. Drain and set aside.

Wash the cucumber and cut into thick slices. Set aside.

Now, process banana, apple, blueberries, and cucumber in a juicer. Transfer to serving glasses and add some ice before serving.

Enjoy!

Nutritional information per serving: Kcal: 348, Protein: 6g, Carbs: 102g, Fats: 1.9g

5.   Watermelon Maple Juice

Ingredients:

1 cup of watermelon, diced

1 tbsp of maple syrup

1 cup plums, pitted and halved

1 large Granny Smith apple, cored

3 oz of water

Preparation:

Cut the watermelon lengthwise. For one cup, you will need about 1 large wedge. Peel and cut into chunks. Remove the seeds and set aside. Reserve the rest of the melon for some other juices.

Wash the plums and cut into halves. Remove the pits and fill the measuring cup. Set aside.

Wash the apple and remove the core. Cut into bite-sized pieces and set aside.

Now, combine watermelon, plums, and apple in a juicer. Process until juiced.

Transfer to serving glasses and stir in the maple syrup and water. Optionally, add some ice or refrigerate before serving.

Enjoy!

Nutritional information per serving: Kcal: 335, Protein: 4.3g, Carbs: 96.8g, Fats: 1.6g

6.   Strawberry Apple Juice

Ingredients:

1 cup strawberries, chopped

1 large Fuji apple, chopped

1 cup pomegranate seeds

1 large orange, peeled

1 cup fresh spinach

2 oz water

Preparation:

Rinse the strawberries under running water and remove the stems. Chop into small pieces and fill the measuring cup. Set aside.

Wash the apple and remove the core. Cut into bite-sized pieces and set aside.

Cut the top of the pomegranate fruit using a sharp knife. Slice down to each of the white membranes inside of the fruit. Pop the seeds into a medium bowl.

Rinse the spinach thoroughly and torn into small pieces. Set aside.

Peel the orange and divide into wedges. Set aside.

Now, process strawberries, apple, pomegranate seeds, spinach, and orange in a juicer. Transfer to serving glasses and stir in the water.

Refrigerate for 10 minutes before serving.

Nutritional information per serving: Kcal: 266, Protein: 6.1g, Carbs: 80.8g, Fats: 2.2g

7.   Mango Plum Juice

Ingredients:

1 cup mango, chopped

3 large plums, pitted

1 large grapefruit, peeled

1 medium-sized green apple, cored

2 oz coconut water

2 tbsp fresh mint, finely chopped

Preparation:

Peel the mango and cut into chunks. Fill the measuring cup and refrigerate the rest for some other juice. Set aside.

Wash the plums and cut in half. Remove the pits and chop into small pieces. Set aside.

Peel the grapefruit and divide into wedges. Cut each wedge in half and set aside.

Wash the apple and remove the core. Cut into bite-sized pieces and set aside.

Now, combine mango, plums, grapefruit, and apple in a juicer. Process until juiced. Transfer to serving glasses and stir in the coconut water.

Add a few ice cubes and garnish with mint.

Serve immediately.

Nutritional information per serving: Kcal: 211, Protein: 9.3g, Carbs: 59.3g, Fats: 1.5g

8.   Melon Agave Juice

Ingredients:

1 cup watermelon, seeded

1 cup honeydew melon, chopped

1 cup pomegranate seeds

1 cup beets, trimmed

2 medium-sized radishes, chopped

1 tbsp agave nectar

Preparation:

Cut the watermelon lengthwise. For one cup, you will need about 1 large wedge. Peel and cut into chunks. Remove the seeds and set aside. Reserve the rest of the melon for some other juices.

Cut the honeydew melon lengthwise in half. Scoop out the seeds using a spoon. Cut into large wedges and peel them. Now, cut into small chunks and place in a bowl. Set aside.

Wash the beets and radishes and trim off the green parts. Chop into small pieces and set aside.

Cut the top of the pomegranate fruit using a sharp knife. Slice down to each of the white membranes inside of the fruit. Pop the seeds into a measuring cup and set aside.

Now, combine watermelon, honeydew melon, beets, and pomegranate seeds in a juicer. Process until juiced.

Transfer to serving glasses and stir in the agave nectar.

Add some ice and serve.

Nutrition information per serving: Kcal: 167, Protein: 13.1g, Carbs: 45.9g, Fats: 1.5g

9.   Cherry Lime Juice

Ingredients:

1 cup honeydew melon, chopped

1 cup sour cherries

1 large lime, peeled

1 large orange, peeled

1 tbsp honey

2 oz coconut water

Preparation:

Rinse the cherries using a colander and cut in half. Remove the pits and set aside.

Peel the lime and cut lengthwise in half. Set aside.

Cut the honeydew melon lengthwise in half. Scoop out the seeds using a spoon. Cut the large wedges and peel them. Cut into small chunks and place in a bowl. Wrap the rest of the melon in a plastic foil and refrigerate.

Peel the orange and divide into wedges. Set aside.

Now, combine cherries, lime, melon, and orange in a juicer. Transfer to serving glasses and stir in the honey and coconut water.

Add some ice and serve immediately.

Nutritional information per serving: Kcal: 276, Protein: 4.2g, Carbs: 78.9g, Fats: 0.7g

10.   Lemon Lime Juice

Ingredients:

2 large lemons, peeled

2 large limes, peeled

3 large oranges, peeled

¼ tsp ginger powder

1 tbsp maple syrup

2 oz water

Preparation:

Peel the lemons and limes and cut lengthwise in half. Set aside.

Peel the oranges and divide into wedges. Cut each wedge in half and set aside.

Now, combine oranges, lemons, and limes in a juicer.

Transfer to serving glasses and stir in the cinnamon, maple syrup, and water.

Add few ice cubes and serve immediately.

Nutrition information per serving: Kcal: 246, Protein: 6.8g, Carbs: 83.1g, Fats: 1.1g

11.   Orange Grape Juice

Ingredients:

1 large blood orange, peeled

1 cup black grapes

1 cup asparagus, trimmed

1 large lemon, peeled

1 large lime, peeled

3 oz water

Preparation:

Peel the orange and divide into wedges. Set aside.

Wash the green grapes under cold running water. Drain water and set aside.

Wash the asparagus and trim off the woody ends. Cut into 1-inch pieces and set aside.

Peel the lemon and lime and cut lengthwise in half. Set aside.

Now, combine orange, grapes, asparagus, lemon, and lime in a juicer. Process until juiced.

Transfer to serving glasses and stir in the water. Add some ice and serve immediately.

Enjoy!

Nutritional information per serving: Kcal: 361, Protein: 5.1g, Carbs: 109g, Fats: 1.5g

12.   Honeydew Cantaloupe Juice

Ingredients:

1 large banana, chopped

¼ tsp cinnamon, ground

1 cup honeydew melon, cubed

1 cup cantaloupe, diced

Preparation:

Peel the banana and cut into small pieces. Set aside.

Cut the melon lengthwise in half. For one cup, cut one large wedge. Peel and chop into small cubes. Remove the seeds and fill the measuring cup. Reserve the rest in the refrigerator.

Cut the cantaloupe in half and scoop out the seeds. Cut and peel two medium wedges. Fill the measuring cup and reserve the rest for later.

Now, combine banana, melon, and cantaloupe in a juicer and process until juiced. Transfer to a serving glass and stir in the cinnamon. Refrigerate for 5 minutes before serving.

Enjoy!

Nutrition information per serving: Kcal: 171, Protein: 3.4g, Carbs: 47.3g, Fats: 0.8g

13.   Watermelon Banana Juice

Ingredients:

1 cup watermelon, diced

1 medium-sized banana, sliced

1 cup celery, chopped

¼ tsp ginger, ground

2 oz water

Preparation:

Cut the watermelon in half. Cut and peel one large wedge. Dice into small pieces and remove the seeds. Fill the measuring cup and wrap the rest of the melon in a plastic foil. Refrigerate for later.

Peel the banana and cut into slices. Set aside.

Wash the celery and cut into bite-sized pieces. Fill the measuring cup and reserve the rest for later.

Now, combine watermelon, banana, and celery in a juicer and process until juiced. Transfer to a serving glass and stir in the water and ginger.

Add some ice and serve immediately.

Enjoy!

Nutrition information per serving: Kcal: 147, Protein: 2.9g, Carbs: 41.4g, Fats: 0.8g

14.   Cinnamon Peach Juice

Ingredients:

3 large peaches, pitted and chopped

1 cup pineapple, peeled and chunked

¼ tsp cinnamon, ground

½ cup cantaloupe, chopped

1 oz water

Preparation:

Wash the peaches and cut in half. Remove the pits and cut into bite-sized pieces. Set aside.

Cut the top of the pineapple and peel it using a sharp paring knife. Peel it all and cut into small pieces. Fill the measuring cup and set aside.

Cut the cantaloupe in half and scoop out the seeds. Cut and peel two medium wedges. Fill the measuring cup and reserve the rest for later.

Now, combine peaches, cantaloupe, and pineapple in a juicer and process until juiced. Transfer to a serving glass and stir in the cinnamon.

Refrigerate for 10 minutes before serving.

Nutrition information per serving: Kcal: 237, Protein: 5.4g, Carbs: 69.1g, Fats: 5.4g

15. Watermelon Swiss Chard Juice

Ingredients:

1 cup watermelon, diced

2 cups Swiss chard, chopped

1 cup pineapple, chunked

¼ tsp ginger, ground

Preparation:

Cut the top of the watermelon. Cut lengthwise in half and then cut one large wedge. Peel it and cut into small cubes. Remove the seeds and fill the measuring cup. Wrap the rest in a plastic foil and refrigerate for later.

Rinse the Swiss chard thoroughly under cold running water. Slightly drain and chop into small pieces. Set aside.

Cut the top of the pineapple and peel it using a sharp paring knife. Peel it all and cut into small pieces. Fill the measuring cup and set aside.

Now, combine watermelon, Swiss chard, and pineapple in a juicer. Process until juiced. Transfer to a serving glass and stir in the ginger.

Add some ice and serve immediately.

Enjoy!

Nutrition information per serving: Kcal: 127, Protein: 3.1g, Carbs: 35.8g, Fats: 0.6g

16.   Mint Apple Juice

Ingredients:

1 cup fresh mint, chopped

1 small Granny Smith's apple, cored

1 large guava, chopped

2 oz water

Preparation:

Wash the mint thoroughly under cold running water. Chop into small pieces and set aside.

Wash the apple and cut in half. Remove the core and cut into bite-sized pieces. Set aside.

Peel the guava and cut lengthwise in half. Scoop out the seeds and chop into small pieces. Set aside.

Now, combine mint, apple, and guava in a juicer and process until juiced. Transfer to a serving glass and stir in the water.

Refrigerate for 5 minutes before serving.

Enjoy!

Nutrition information per serving: Kcal: 288, Protein: 4.4g, Carbs: 91.7g, Fats: 1.6g

17.   Apple Pomegranate Juice

Ingredients:

1 large Granny Smith's apple, chopped

1 cup of pomegranate seeds

1 large peach, pitted and halved

3 oz of water

1 tbsp agave nectar

Preparation:

Wash the apple and cut in half. Remove the core and cut into bite-sized pieces. Set aside.

Cut the top of the pomegranate fruit using a sharp knife. Slice down to each of the white membranes inside of the fruit. Pop the seeds into measuring cup and set aside.

Wash the peach and cut in half. Remove the pit and cut into small pieces. Set aside.

Now, combine apple, pomegranate seeds, and peach in a juicer and process until juiced.

Transfer to serving glasses and stir in the water and agave nectar.

Add some ice and serve!

Nutrition information per serving: Kcal: 212, Protein: 3.9g, Carbs: 61g, Fats: 1.8g

18.   Cucumber Mango Juice

Ingredients:

1 cup blueberries

1 cup cucumber, sliced

1 cup mango, chunked

1 medium-sized green apple, cored

2 oz water

Preparation:

Peel the cucumber and cut into slices. Fill the measuring cup and reserve the rest for later.

Wash the mango and cut into chunks. Fill the measuring cup and reserve the rest for some other juice. Set aside.

Rinse the blueberries under cold running water using a colander. Drain and set aside.

Wash the apple and remove the core. Cut into bite-sized pieces and set aside.

Now, combine cucumber, mango, blueberries, and apple in a juicer. Process until juiced.

Transfer to a serving glass and stir in the water. Add some ice before serving and enjoy!

Nutrition information per serving: Kcal: 178, Protein: 5.8g, Carbs: 61.5g, Fats: 1.1g

19.   Zucchini Grape Juice

Ingredients:

1 small zucchini, chopped

1 cup black grapes

1 medium-sized pear, chopped

¼ tsp cinnamon, ground

2 oz water

Preparation:

Peel the zucchini and cut into bite-sized cubes. Set aside.

Wash the grapes and fill the measuring cup. Set aside.

Wash the pear and cut in half. Remove the core and cut into small pieces. Set aside.

Now, combine zucchini, grapes, and pear in a juicer. Process until juiced. Transfer to a serving glass and stir in the cinnamon and water.

Add some crushed ice and serve immediately.

Enjoy!

Nutrition information per serving: Kcal: 153, Protein: 2.6 g, Carbs: 46.6g, Fats: 0.9g

20.   Apple Cucumber Juice

Ingredients:

1 large Granny Smith's apple, chopped

1 large cucumber, sliced

2 large honeydew melon wedges

2 oz of water

Preparation:

Wash and peel the apple. Cut in half and remove the core. Cut into bite-sized pieces and set aside.

Peel the cucumber. Cut into thin slices and set aside.

Cut the honeydew melon lengthwise in half. Scoop out the seeds using a spoon. Cut two large wedges and peel them. Cut into small chunks and fill the measuring cup. Wrap the rest of the melon in a plastic foil and refrigerate.

Now, combine apple, cucumber, and honeydew melon in a juicer. Process until juiced. Transfer to serving glasses and stir in the water.

Add some ice before serving and enjoy!

Nutrition information per serving: Kcal: 241, Protein: 4.6g, Carbs: 68.1g, Fats: 1.2g

21.   Peach Lemon Juice

Ingredients:

1 large peach, pitted and halved

1 large lemon, peeled

1 large orange, peeled

1 medium-sized cucumber, sliced

1 cup pomegranate seeds

2 oz water

1 tbsp of maple syrup

Preparation:

Wash the peach and cut in half. Remove the pit and cut into small pieces. Set aside.

Peel the lemon and cut lengthwise in half. Set aside.

Peel the orange and divide into wedges. Set aside.

Wash the cucumber and cut into thin slices. Set aside.

Cut the top of the pomegranate fruit using a sharp knife. Slice down to each of the white membranes inside of the fruit. Pop the seeds into measuring cup and set aside.

Now, combine peach, lemon, orange, cucumber, and pomegranate seeds in a juicer. Process until juiced.

Transfer to serving glasses and stir in the water and maple syrup.

Refrigerate for 5 minutes before serving.

Nutrition information per serving: Kcal: 265, Protein: 5.6g, Carbs: 63.7g, Fats: 1.8g

22.   Radish Apple Juice

Ingredients:

1 cup radishes, chopped

1 medium-sized apple, peeled and wedged

1 large orange, peeled

1 cup Romain lettuce, torn

1 cup watercress, torn

1 tbsp honey

Preparation:

Wash the radishes and trim off the green parts. Cut into small pieces and fill the measuring cup. Set aside.

Wash the apple and cut in half. Remove the core and chop into small pieces. Set aside.

Peel the orange and divide into wedges. Set aside.

Rinse the lettuce and watercress using a large colander. Drain and torn with hands.

Now, combine radishes, apple, orange, lettuce, and watercress in a juicer. Process until juiced.

Transfer to serving glasses and add some ice before serving.

Enjoy!

Nutrition information per serving: Kcal: 150, Protein: 7.3g, Carbs: 53.4g, Fats: 0.8g

23. Apple Beet Juice

Ingredients:

1 large Honeycrisp apple, cored

2 medium-sized beets, trimmed

1 large cucumber, sliced

1 whole lime, peeled

¼ tsp ginger powder

Preparation:

Wash the apple and remove the core. Cut into bite-sized pieces and set aside.

Wash the beets and trim off the green ends. Save it for another juice. Cut the beet into small pieces. Set aside.

Wash the cucumber and cut it into thick slices. Set aside.

Peel the lime and cut into quarters. Set aside.

Now, process apple, beets, cucumber, and lime in a juicer. Transfer to serving glasses and add some ice before serving.

Enjoy!

Nutrition information per serving: Kcal: 109, Protein: 2.8g, Carbs: 33.6g, Fats: 0.7g

24.   Apricot Mango Juice

Ingredients:

1 cup apricots, sliced

1 cup mango, chopped

½ cup coconut water

1 tbsp maple syrup

Preparation:

Wash the apricots and cut in half. Remove the pits and chop into small pieces. Set aside.

Peel the mango and cut into small chunks. Fill the measuring cup and rserve the rest in the refrigerator.

Now, combine apricots, mango, and coconut water in a juicer. Process until juiced.

Transfer to serving glasses and stir in the maple syrup.

Add few ice cubes and serve immediately.

Nutrition information per serving: Kcal: 155, Protein: 3.6g, Carbs: 43g, Fats: 1.2g

25.   Basil Raspberry Juice

Ingredients:

1 cup fresh basil, torn

2 cups raspberries

1 cup beets, chopped

1 large Granny Smith's apple, cored

1 whole lemon, peeled

3 oz water

Preparation:

Wash the basil thoroughly under cold running water and torn with hands. Set aside.

Wash the raspberries under cold running water using a colander. Drain and set aside.

Wash the beets and trim off the green ends. Cut into small pieces and fill the measuring cup. Reserve the greens for some other juice.

Wash the apple and cut in half. Remove the core and cut into bite-sized pieces. Set aside.

Peel the lemon and cut lengthwise in half. Set aside.

Now, combine basil, raspberries, beets, apple, and lemon in a juicer. Process until well juiced.

Stir in the water and refrigerate for 10-15 minutes before serving.

Enjoy!

Nutrition information per serving: Kcal: 218, Protein: 7.5g, Carbs: 76.4g, Fats: 2.5g

26.   Strawberry Grapefruit Juice

Ingredients:

2 large strawberries, chopped

2 large grapefruits, peeled

1 large Red Delicious apple, cored

1 small ginger knob, peeled

2 oz coconut water

Preparation:

Rinse the strawberries using a colander. Remove the green stems and cut into small pieces. Set aside.

Peel the grapefruits and divide into wedges. Cut each wedge in half and set aside.

Wash the apple and cut in half. Remove the core and cut into bite-sized pieces. Set aside.

Peel the ginger knob and set aside.

Now, combine strawberries, grapefruit, apple, and ginger in a juicer. Process until well juiced.

Transfer to serving glasses and stir in the coconut water. Refrigerate for 5 minutes before serving.

Enjoy!

Nutrition information per serving: Kcal: 302, Protein: 4.8g, Carbs: 86.3g, Fats: 1.7g

27.   Apricot Raspberry Juice

Ingredients:

3 whole apricots, pitted

1 cup fresh blackberries

1 cup fresh raspberries

1 large Fuji apple, cored

3 large carrots, peeled and sliced

Preparation:

Combine blackberries and raspberries in a colander. Rinse well under cold running water and slightly drain. Set aside.

Wash the apricots and cut in half. Remove the pits and cut into bite-sized pieces. Set aside.

Wash the apple and cut in half. Remove the core and cut into small pieces.

Wash and peel the carrots. Cut into thin slices and set aside.

Now, combine apricots, raspberries, blackberries, apple, and carrots in a juicer. Process until well juiced and transfer to serving glasses. Stir in the water and refrigerate for 5 minutes before serving.

Enjoy!

Nutrition information per serving: Kcal: 301, Protein: 7.6g, Carbs: 97.4g, Fats: 2.9g

28.   Mint Strawberry Juice

Ingredients:

1 cup fresh mint, chopped

1 cup strawberries, chopped

1 cup avocado, pitted

1 large Honeycrisp apple, cored and chopped

1 large lemon, peeled

1 large cucumber, sliced

Preparation:

Wash the mint thoroughly and torn with hands. Set aside.

Wash the strawberries and cut into small pieces. Set aside.

Peel the avocado and cut lengthwise in half. Remove the pit and cut into chunks and fill the measuring cup. Reserve the rest for later.

Wash the apple and cut in half. Remove the core and cut into bite-sized pieces. Set aside.

Peel the lemon and cut lengthwise in half. Set aside.

Peel the cucumber and cut into thin slices. Set aside.

Now, combine mint, strawberries, avocado, lemon, and cucumber in a juicer. Process until juiced. Transfer to serving glasses and stir in the water.

Add some ice before serving.

Nutrition information per serving: Kcal: 376, Protein: 8.1g, Carbs: 67.8g, Fats: 23.3g

29.   Orange Cranberry Juice

Ingredients:

1 large orange, peeled

1 cup fresh cranberries

1 cup fresh strawberries

2 oz coconut water

Preparation:

Combine cranberries and strawberries in a colander. Rinse under cold running water. Drain and set aside.

Peel the orange and divide into wedges. Cut each wedge in half and set aside.

Combine cranberries, strawberries, and orange in a juicer. Process until juiced.

Transfer to serving glasses and stir in the coconut water.

Add some ice and serve immediately.

Nutrition information per serving: Kcal: 137, Protein: 3.2g, Carbs: 46.6g, Fats: 0.8g

30.   Grape Beet Juice

Ingredients:

1 cup black grapes

1 cup beets, trimmed and sliced

1 large blood orange, peeled

1 whole apricot, pitted

1 tbsp coconut water

Preparation:

Rinse the grapes and remove the stems. Set aside.

Wash the beets and trim off the green parts. Cut into thin slices and fill the measuring cup. Reserve the rest for later.

Peel the orange and divide into wedges. Cut each wedge in half and set aside.

Wash the apricot and cut lengthwise in half. Remove the pit and cut into small pieces. Set aside.

Now, combine grapes, beets, orange, and apricots in a juicer and process until well juiced. Transfer to a serving glass and stir in the coconut water.

Add some ice and serve immediately.

Nutrition information per serving: Kcal: 184, Protein: 4.9g, Carbs: 54.3g, Fats: 0.9g

31. Banana Apricot Juice

Ingredients:

1 medium-sized banana, sliced

3 whole apricots, chopped

1 medium-sized celery stalk, chopped

1 small Fuji apple, chopped

1 tsp maple syrup

1 oz water

Preparation:

Peel the banana and cut into small chunks. Set aside.

Rinse the apricots and cut in half. Remove the pits and cut into bite-sized pieces. Set aside.

Rinse the celery stalk and cut into bite-sized pieces. Set aside.

Wash the apple and cut in half. Remove the core and cut into bite-sized pieces. Set aside.

Now, combine banana, apricots, celery, and apple in a juicer and process until juiced. Transfer to a serving glass and stir in the maple syrup and add few ice cubes.

Serve immediately.

Nutrition information per serving: Kcal: 185, Protein: 3.6g, Carbs: 68.8g, Fats: 1.6g

32.   Beet Carrot Juice

Ingredients:

1 cup beets, trimmed

1 large carrot, sliced

1 cup avocado, chopped

1 small ginger knob, 1-inch thick

2 oz water

Preparation:

Trim off the green parts of the beets. Peel and cut into thin slices. Fill the measuring cup and reserve the remaining beet in the refrigerator.

Wash and peel the carrot. Cut into bite-sized pieces and set aside.

Peel the avocado and cut lengthwise in half. Remove the pit and cut into bite-sized pieces. Fill the measuring cup and reserve the rest in the refrigerator.

Peel the ginger knob and cut into small pieces. Set aside.

Now, combine beets, carrot, avocado, and ginger in a juicer. Process until well juiced and transfer to a serving glass. Stir in the and water and refrigerate for 5-10 minutes before serving.

Enjoy!

Nutrition information per serving: Kcal: 265, Protein: 5.9g, Carbs: 33.4g, Fats: 21.8g

33.   Cantaloupe Orange Juice

Ingredients:

1 cup cantaloupe, chopped

1 large orange, peeled

1 whole plum, chopped

1 cup fresh mint, torn

¼ tsp ginger, ground

Preparation:

Cut the cantaloupe in half. Scoop out the seeds and flesh. Cut and peel one large wedge. Chop into chunks and fill the measuring cup. Reserve the rest of the cantaloupe in a refrigerator.

Peel the orange and divide into wedges. Cut each wedge in half and set aside.

Wash the plum and cut in half. Remove the pit and chop into small pieces. Set aside.

Rinse the mint thoroughly under cold running water. Torn into small pieces and set aside.

Now, combine cantaloupe, orange, plum, and mint in a juicer and process until juiced. Transfer to a serving glass and stir in the ginger.

Add some ice and serve immediately.

Enjoy!

Nutrition information per serving: Kcal: 151, Protein: 4.4g, Carbs: 45.6g, Fats: 0.9g

34. Apple Strawberry Juice

Ingredients:

1 cup blackberries

1 medium-sized Honeycrisp apple, cored and chopped

1 cup strawberries, chopped

1 large pear, chopped

¼ tsp cinnamon, ground

1 oz water

Preparation:

Wash the apple and cut lengthwise in half. Remove the core and chop into bite-sized pieces. Set aside.

Rinse strawberries and remove the stems. Cut into small pieces and fill the measuring cup. Reserve the rest in the refrigerator.

Wash the blackberries using a colander. Drain and set aside.

Wash the pear and cut in half. Remove the core and cut into small pieces. Set aside.

Now, combine apple, strawberries, blackberries, and pear in a juicer and process until well juiced. Transfer to a serving glass and stir in the cinnamon.

Refrigerate for 10 minutes before serving.

Enjoy!

Nutrition information per serving: Kcal: 246, Protein: 4.2g, Carbs: 82.1g, Fats: 1.7g

35.   Pomegranate Lemon Juice

Ingredients:

1 cup pomegranate seeds

1 whole lemon, peeled

1 cup fresh spinach, torn

2 oz water

Preparation:

Cut the top of the pomegranate fruit using a sharp paring knife. Slice down to each of the white membranes inside of the fruit. Pop the seeds into a measuring cup and set aside.

Peel the lemon and cut lengthwise in half. Set aside.

Rinse the spinach thoroughly under cold running water. Drain and torn into small pieces. Set aside.

Now, combine pomegranate seeds, spinach, and lemon in a juicer. Process until well juiced.

Transfer to a serving glass and stir in the water. Add some ice and serve immediately.

Enjoy!

Nutrition information per serving: Kcal: 195, Protein: 10.2g, Carbs: 56.1g, Fats: 2.1g

36.   Apple Guava Juice

Ingredients:

1 small Granny Smith's apple, cored and chopped

1 whole guava, chunked

1 cup strawberries, chopped

1 whole lemon, peeled and halved

¼ tsp cinnamon, ground

2 oz water

Preparation:

Wash the apple and cut lengthwise in half. Remove the core and cut into bite-sized pieces. Set aside.

Peel the guava and cut in half. Scoop out the seeds and wash it. Cut into small chunks and set aside.

Wash the strawberries and remove the stems. Cut into small pieces and fill the measuring cup. Reserve the rest in the refrigerator. Set aside.

Peel the lemon and cut lengthwise in half. Set aside.

Now, combine apple, guava, strawberries, and lemon in a juicer and process until juiced. Transfer to a serving glass and stir in the cinnamon and water.

Refrigerate for 5 minutes before serving.

Enjoy!

Nutrition information per serving: Kcal: 136, Protein: 3.6g, Carbs: 43.9g, Fats: 1.3g

37.   Banana Blueberry Juice

Ingredients:

1 large banana, peeled

1 cup blueberries

1 cup cherries, pitted

1 whole lemon, peeled

1 small Fuji apple, cored

¼ tsp cinnamon powder

Preparation:

Peel the banana and cut into small chunks. Set aside.

Rinse the blueberries using a large colander. Drain and set aside.

Wash the cherries and cut in half. Remove the pits and stems. Set aside.

Peel the lemon and cut lengthwise in half. Set aside.

Wash the apple and cut lengthwise in half. Remove the core and cut into small pieces. Set aside.

Now, combine banana, blueberries, cherries, lemon, and apple in a juicer and process until juiced. Transfer to a serving glass and stir in the cinnamon.

Add some ice and serve immediately.

Nutrition information per serving: Kcal: 340, Protein: 5.5g, Carbs: 102g, Fats: 1.7g

38. Apricot Banana Juice

Ingredients:

3 whole apricots, chopped

1 large banana, chunked

2 whole kiwis, peeled and halved

1 medium-sized Honeycrisp apple, cored and chopped

Preparation:

Wash the apricots and cut in half. Remove the pits and cut into small pieces. Set aside.

Peel the banana and cut into small chunks. Set aside.

Peel the kiwi and cut lengthwise in half. Set aside.

Wash the apple and cut lengthwise in half. Remove the core and cut into bite-sized pieces. Set aside.

Now, combine apricots, banana, kiwi, and apple in a juicer and process until juiced. Transfer to a serving glass and add some ice.

Serve immediately.

Nutrition information per serving: Kcal: 313, Protein: 5.4g, Carbs: 91g, Fats: 1.9g

39.   Pineapple Lime Juice

Ingredients:

1 cup pineapple, chunked

1 whole lime, peeled

1 cup blackberries

1 large banana, sliced

2 oz water

Preparation:

Using a sharp paring knife, cut the top of the pineapple. Gently remove all hard skin and slice it into thin slices. Fill the measuring cup and reserve the rest for later.

Peel the lime and cut lengthwise in half. Set aside.

Place the blackberries in a small colander and wash under cold running water. Slightly drain and set aside.

Peel the banana and cut into thin slices. Set aside.

Now, combine pineapple, lime, blackberries, and banana in a juicer. Process until well juiced. Transfer to a serving glass and add some ice before serving.

Enjoy!

Nutrition information per serving: Kcal: 222, Protein: 4.5g, Carbs: 70.2g, Fats: 1.4g

40.   Asparagus Orange Juice

Ingredients:

1 cup asparagus, trimmed

3 medium-sized blood oranges, peeled and wedged

1 large Fuji apple, cored

¼ tsp ginger, ground

2 oz water

Preparation:

Rinse the asparagus thoroughly under cold running water using a colander. Trim off the woody ends. Cut into small pieces and set aside.

Peel the oranges and divide into wedges. Set aside.

Wash the apple and remove the core. Cut into bite-sized pieces and set aside.

Now, combine asparagus, oranges, and apple in a juicer and process until juiced. Transfer to serving glasses and stir in the ginger and water.

Refrigerate for 10 minutes before serving.

Nutrition information per serving: Kcal: 316, Protein: 9.1g, Carbs: 98.1g, Fats: 1.2g

41.   Broccoli Lemon Juice

Ingredients:

1 cup broccoli, chopped

1 whole lemon, peeled

1 large cucumber, sliced

1 cup avocado, chopped

1 large lime, peeled

1 oz water

Preparation:

Rinse the broccoli under running water. Chop into small pieces and fill the measuring cup. Set aside.

Peel the lemon and lime. Cut lengthwise in half. Set aside.

Peel the cucumber and cut in thick slices. Set aside.

Peel the avocado and cut in half. Remove the pit and cut into chunks. Set aside.

Now, combine broccoli, lemon, cucumber, avocado, and lime in a juicer. Process until juiced. Transfer to serving glasses and stir in the water.

Add some ice and serve immediately.

Nutritional information per serving: Kcal: 281, Protein: 8.3g, Carbs: 38.8g, Fats: 22.8g

42.   Orange Cucumber Juice

Ingredients:

2 large oranges, peeled

1 large cucumber, peeled

1 cup broccoli, chopped

1 large carrot, sliced

1 oz water

Preparation:

Peel the oranges and divide into wedges. Set aside.

Wash the cucumber and cut into thin slices. Set aside.

Wash the broccoli and trim off the outer leaves. Cut into small pieces and fill the measuring cup. Reserve the rest in the refrigerator.

Now, combine oranges, cucumber, broccoli, and carrot in a juicer and process until juiced.

Transfer to a serving glass and stir in the water.

Add few ice cubes and serve immediately!

Nutritional information per serving: Kcal: 68, Protein: 2.3g, Carbs: 19.7g, Fats: 0.1g

43.　Apple Lemon Juice

Ingredients:

1 large Granny Smith's apple, cored

1 whole lemon, peeled

3 medium-sized celery stalks, chopped

½ cup freh cilantro, chopped

¼ tsp ginger powder

1 tsp maple syrup

Preparation:

Wash the apple and cut in half. Remove the core and cut into small pieces. Set aside.

Peel the lemon and cut lengthwise in half. Set aside.

Rinse the celery and chop into small pieces. Set aside.

Now, combine apple, lemon, celery, and cilantro in a juicer. Process until juiced. Transfer to serving glasses and stir in the ginger and maple syrup.

Add few ice cubes and serve immediately.

Nutritional information per serving: Kcal: 153, Protein: 2.3g, Carbs: 38.4g, Fats: 0.2g

44.   Banana Pomegranate Juice

Ingredients:

1 large banana, chunked

1 cup pomegranate seeds

1 medium-sized Honeycrisp apple, cored

1 tbsp agave nectar

1 oz water

Preparation:

Peel the banana and cut into small chunks. Set aside.

Cut the top of the pomegranate fruit using a sharp paring knife. Slice down to each of the white membranes inside of the fruit. Pop the seeds into a measuring cup and set aside.

Wash the apple and cut lengthwise in half. Remove the core and cut into bite-sized pieces. Set aside.

Now, combine banana, pomegranate seeds, and apple in a juicer. Process until juiced. Transfer to a serving glass and stir in the agave nectar and water.

Serve cold.

Nutrition information per serving: Kcal: 243, Protein: 3.6g, Carbs: 70.1g, Fats: 1.8g

45.   Artichoke Cherry Juice

Ingredients:

1 cup artichokes, chopped

1 cup fresh cherries, pitted

1 whole lemon, peeled

1 medium-sized Fuji apple, cored

¼ tsp cinnamon, ground

Preparation:

Rinse the artichoke and trim off the outer, hard leaves. Cut into bite-sized pieces and fill the measuring cup. Reserve the rest in the refrigerator.

Rinse the cherries under running water using a colander. Cut each in half and remove the pits. Set aside.

Peel the lemon and cut lengthwise in half. Set aside.

Wash the apple and cut lengthwise in half. Remove the core and cut into bite-sized pieces. Set aside.

Now, combine artichoke, cherries, lemon, and apple in a juicer and process until juiced. Transfer to a serving glass and stir in the cinnamon.

Refrigerate for 10 minutes before serving.

Nutrition information per serving: Kcal: 205, Protein: 7.2g, Carbs: 66.2g, Fats: 0.9g

46.   Carrot Celery Juice

Ingredients:

1 medium-sized carrot, sliced

1 cup celery, chopped

1 small Roma tomato, chopped

1 cup fresh spinach, torn

¼ tsp salt

¼ tsp balsamic vinegar

Preparation:

Wash and peel the carrot. Cut into thin slices and set aside.

Wash the celery and chop into small pieces. Set aside.

Wash the tomato and place in a small bowl. Cut into bite-sized pieces. Make sure to reserve the tomato juice while cutting. Set aside.

Wash the spinach thoroughly under cold running water. Torn into small pieces and set aside.

Now, combine carrot, celery, tomato, and spinach in a juicer. Process until juiced. Transfer to a serving glass and stir in the salt, vinegar, and reserved tomato juice.

Refrigerate for 20 minutes before serving.

Nutrition information per serving: Kcal: 72, Protein: 8.4g, Carbs: 21.2g, Fats: 1.4g

47.   Apple Watermelon Juice

Ingredients:

1 medium-sized Granny Smith's apple, cored and chopped

1 cup watermelon, cubed

1 large peach, pitted and chopped

1 banana, peeled and sliced

¼ tsp cinnamon, ground

Preparation:

Wash the apple and cut in half. Remove the core and cut into bite-sized pieces. Set aside.

Cut the watermelon in half. Cut one large wedge and wrap the rest in a plastic foil and refrigerate. Peel the slice and cut into small cubes. Remove the pits and fill the measuring cup. Set aside.

Wash the peach and cut lengthwise in half. Remove the pit and chop into bite-sized pieces. Set aside.

Peel the banana and cut into thin slices. Set aside.

Now, combine watermelon, peach, apple, and banana in a juicer and process until juiced. Transfer to a serving glass and stir in the cinnamon.

Add some ice and serve immediately!

Nutrition information per serving: Kcal: 260, Protein: 4.4g, Carbs: 73.9g, Fats: 1.3g

48.   Grape Spinach Juice

Ingredients:

1 cup black grapes

1 cup fresh spinach, torn

1 cup broccoli, chopped

1 small Granny Smith's apple, cored

1 tbsp fresh mint, finely chopped

Preparation:

Rinse the grapes under running water and remove the stems. Set aside.

Using a large colander, rinse the broccoli and spinach under cold running water. Drain and torn the spinach in small pieces. Trim off the outer leaves of the broccoli and cut into small pieces. Fill the measuring cups and set aside.

Wash the apple and cut lengthwise in half. Remove the core and cut into bite-sized pieces. Set aside.

Now, combine grapes, spinach, broccoli, and apple in a juicer and process until well juiced. Transfer to a serving glass and sprinkle with some fresh mint.

Refrigerate for 10 minutes before serving.

Nutrition information per serving: Kcal: 176, Protein: 9.8g, Carbs: 49.5g, Fats:1.7g

49.   Avocado Lettuce Juice

Ingredients:

1 cup avocado, chunked

1 cup Iceberg lettuce, chopped

1 large carrot, chopped

1 cup collard greens, torn

1 cucumber, sliced

¼ tsp ginger, ground

Preparation:

Peel the avocado and cut lengthwise in half. Remove the pit and cut into small chunks. Fill the measuring cup and reserve the rest in the refrigerator.

Wash and peel the carrot. Cut into thin slices and set aside.

Place lettuce and collard greens in a large colander. Rinse well thoroughly under cold running water. Drain and chop into small pieces. Set aside.

Wash the cucumber and cut into thin slices. Fill the measuring cup and reserve the rest for later. Set aside.

Now, combine avocado, lettuce, carrot, collard greens, and cucumber in a juicer and process until juiced. Transfer to a serving glass and stir in the ginger.

Refrigerate for 5 minutes before serving.

Nutrition information per serving: Kcal: 271, Protein: 7.3g, Carbs: 34.1g, Fats: 22.8g

MEALS

1.   Potato Pie

Ingredients:

- 3 medium-sized potatoes, peeled and shredded
- 6 oz of cheddar cheese, crumbled
- 1 cup of skim milk
- 1 medium-sized onion, diced
- ½ tsp of salt
- ¼ tsp of black pepper, ground
- 2 large eggs
- 1 tbsp of vegetable oil

Preparation:

Preheat the oven to 350°F.

Combine potatoes and cheese in a large bowl. Stir well and spread over a previously greased baking sheet. Press equally to make a fine pie crust.

Combine eggs and onion and stir well. Pour over the crust and bake for 45 minutes. Remove from the pan if a knife inserted in the center comes out clean. Set aside to cool for 5 minutes.

Top with some extra shredded cheese for extra calcium and serve!

Nutrition information per serving: Kcal: 209, Protein: 17.6g, Carbs: 26.8g, Fats: 10.3g

2. Berry Mix Smoothie

Ingredients:

- ¼ cup of strawberries, chopped
- ¼ cup of frozen raspberries
- ¼ cup of frozen blueberries
- 1 tbsp of honey
- 1 tsp of lemon juice

Preparation:

Combine all ingredients in a blender and blend until smooth. Transfer to a serving glass.

Serve with ice cubes or refrigerate for an hour before serving.

Nutrition information per serving: Kcal: 163, Protein: 2.1g, Carbs: 42.7g, Fats: 0.2g

3.   Perch with Pasta

Ingredients:

- 1 lb of perch, boneless and cubed (can be replaced with other white fish)
- 8 oz of pasta
- 2 cups of tomato sauce
- 2 tbsp of olive oil
- 2 tbsp of lemon juice
- 1 tsp of balsamic vinegar
- 1 garlic clove, crushed
- 1 tsp of vegetable mix seasoning
- 2 tbsp of fresh parsley, finely chopped

Preparation:

Use the package instructions to prepare the pasta. Drain well and set aside.

Heat up the oil in a large skillet over a medium-high temperature. Add garlic and saute for 2 minutes, or until translucent. Add chopped fish and season with pepper, vegetable seasoning mix, and lemon juice. Cook until fish is nearly done. Pour in the tomato sauce and reduce temperature to low. Simmer for 10-15 minutes. Remove from the heat.

Add pasta to the skillet. Give it a good stir to coat pasta with sauce and juices. Drizzle with vinegar and fresh parsley. Serve.

Nutrition information per serving: Kcal: 277, Protein: 23.9g, Carbs: 22.5g, Fats: 10.2g

4.   Spinach Salad

Ingredients:

- 8 oz of spinach, roughly chopped
- 8 oz of strawberries, halved
- 1 medium-sized red onion, sliced
- 1 medium-sized cucumber, sliced
- 2 tbsp of almonds, chopped
- 2 tbsp of lemon juice
- 1 tbsp of apple cider vinegar
- 1 tbsp of olive oil
- 1 tbsp of honey
- ¼ tsp of salt

Preparation:

Combine lemon juce, vinegar, oil, honey, and salt in a mixing bowl. Stir well and set aside to allow flavors to mingle.

Combine spinach, strawberries, onion, cucumber, and

almonds in a large salad bowl. Drizzle with dressing and toss well before serving.

Nutrition information per serving: Kcal: 142, Protein: 4.3g, Carbs: 21.7g, Fats: 7.2g

5.   Chocolate Cranberry Smoothie

Ingredients:

- ¼ cup of chocolate chips

- ½ cup of skim milk

- 6 oz of vanilla yogurt

- 1 cup of fresh cranberries

Preparation:

Combine all ingredients in a food processor. Blend for one minute or until smooth. Transfer to a serving glasses and add some ice. You can use frozen berries instead of ice.

Top with shredded dark chocolate.

Nutrition information per serving: Kcal: 461, Protein: 13.1g, Carbs: 71.7g, Fats: 10.3g

6. Banana Peppers

Ingredients:

- 10 banana sweet peppers
- 1 lb of ground lean beaf
- ¼ cup of all-purpose flour
- ½ cup of Swiss cheese, shredded
- 1 medium-sized onion, chopped
- 1 tsp of vegetable oil
- 1 large egg
- ¼ tsp of black pepper, ground

Preparation:

Preheat the oven to 350°F.

Heat the oil in a large frying pan over a medium-high temperature. Add the onion, and stir-fry until golden brown. Add the meat and cook until nicely brown. Stir in the cheese and cook for 2 minutes more. Remove from the heat and set aside to cool for a while.

Clean the peppers, removing top and bottom parts. Stuff the peppers with meat mixture.

Beat the egg and combine with pepper in a mixing bowl. Dip the stuffed peppers in egg mixture. Coat with flour, dip in egg, and coat again.

Spray the baking sheet with some vegetable oil and place the peppers. Bake for about 20 minutes.

Top with sour cream, but this is, however optional.

Nutrition information per serving: Kcal: 385, Protein: 29.3g, Carbs: 18.3g, Fats: 15.4g

7. Potato Soup

Ingredients:

- 3 medium-sized potatoes, peeled and mashed
- 3 tbsp of Parmesan cheese, shredded
- ½ cup of celery, finely chopped
- 1 tsp of fresh parsley, finely chopped
- 1 medium-sized onion, sliced
- 1 medium-sized carrot, sliced
- 12 oz of chicken broth
- 4 oz of milk, non-fat
- 1 tbsp of all-purpose flour
- 1 tsp of salt

Preparation:

Combine all ingredients in a slow cooker, except cheese and milk. Cover with a lid and cook for 7 hours on a medium heat.

Combine flour and milk in a mixing bowl and whisk well.

Pour it into the cooker and sprinkle with shredded cheese. Cook for another 20 minutes without lid.

Serve warm.

Nutrition information per serving: Kcal: 324, Protein: 5.3g, Carbs: 28.3g, Fats: 7.3g

8.   Salmon Croquettes

Ingredients:

- 12 oz of wild salmon, skinless and boneless
- 3 tbsp of breadcrumbs
- 2 grain bread slices
- 5 tbsp of mayonnaise
- 1 medium-sized onion, chopped
- 1 small bell pepper, chopped
- ½ tsp of salt
- ¼ tsp of black pepper, ground

Preparation:

Preheat the oven to 400°F.

Combine all ingredients except breadcrumbs in a large bowl. Stir well to combine. Using hands, shape the croquettes and coat well with breadcrumbs.

Line some baking paper over a baking sheet and place the croquettes. Bake for about 20 minutes and remove from the oven.

Serve warm.

Nutrition information per serving: Kcal: 137, Protein: 15.3g, Carbs: 10.4g, Fats: 11.3g

9.   Pumpkin muffins

Ingredients:

- 2 cups of pumpkin pie mix

- 1 cup of flour, whole wheat

- ¼ cup of milk, low-fat

- 2 tbsp of oat meal

- 2 large eggs

- ½ cup of applesauce

- ¼ cup of raisins

- ½ cup of walnuts, finely chopped

- 1 tsp of baking powder

- 1 tsp of vanilla extract

- 1 tbsp of butter

- 1 tsp of baking soda

Preparation:

Preheat the oven to 350°F.

Mix flour, baking powder, oats and soda in a large mixing bowl. Add pumpkin mix and stir all well together to combine. Set aside.

Now, combine raisins, walnuts, milk, butter, applesauce, and vanilla extract in a separate bowl. Stir well to combine. Now, combine both mixtures and give it a good stir.

Fill up lightly greased muffin molds with batter and put it in the oven.

Bake for 25 minutes and remove from the oven. Let it cool for about 15 minutes and serve.

Top with chocolate or cinnamon sprinkle.

Nutrition information per serving: Kcal: 172, Protein: 2.4g, Carbs: 38.8g, Fats: 8.9g

10. Smoked Gouda Omelet

Ingredients:

- 3 tbsp of smoked gouda cheese, shredded
- 1 free-range egg
- 4 egg whites
- 1 medium-sized onion, sliced
- 1 tsp of yellow mustard
- 2 tbsp of skim milk
- 2 tsp of vegetable oil

Preparation:

Preheat 1 teaspoon of oil in a large frying pan over a medium-high temperature. add the onion and stir-fry until translucent. You can add a tablespoon of water to get more juice. Transfer the onion to a mixing bowl and stir in the mustard. Set aside.

Preheat remaining oil over a medium temperature. Meanwhile, combine milk, egg, and whites. Whisk well and pour the mixture into the skillet. Cook until eggs are nearly done. Spread the onion and gouda cheese over one half of the omelet. Flip over another half and cook for 2minutes more. Remove from the heat and cut into portions. Serve.

Nutrition information per serving: Kcal: 201, Protein: 13.5g, Carbs: 18.7g, Fats: 8.8g

11.   Leek and Carrot Soup

Ingredients:

- 1 cup of leeks, chopped

- 1 medium-sized potato, peeled and sliced

- 2 medium-sized carrots, sliced

- 1 cup of chicken broth

- 2 cups of skim milk

- 1 cup of corn, frozen

- 2 tbsp of fresh parsley, finely chopped

- ½ tsp of salt

- ¼ tsp of black pepper, ground

Preparation:

Mix together leeks, potato, carrots in a large pot. Pour in vegetable broth and sprinkle with salt and pepper. Cover with a lid and cook for about 10-15 minutes, or until fork-tender.

Now, add corn and milk and simmer for 5 minutes. Remove from the heat transfer to a serving bowls.

Sprinkle with parsley and serve.

Nutrition information per serving: Kcal: 241, Protein: 13.2g, Carbs: 43.6g, Fats: 8.3g

12.   Catfish with Pecans

Ingredients:

- 1 lb of catfish fillets
- 1 cup of pecans, ground
- ½ cup of skim milk
- 1 tbsp of olive oil
- 6 tbsp of Dijon mustard
- 1 tbsp of lemon juice
- 3 small potatoes, peeled and cubed

Preparation:

Preheat the oven to 400°F.

Put potatoes in a pot of boiling water. Sprinkle with vegetable seasoning mix and cook until fork-tender. Drain and set aside to cool for a while.

Combine mustard and milk in a mixing bowl. Dipp fish fillets in the mixture then coat with pecans. Place the fillets on a greased baking sheet and put it in the oven. Bake for 10-12 minutes. remove from the oven and serve with potatoes.

Drizzle potatoes with lemon juice and serve.

Nutrition information per serving: Kcal: 438, Protein: 24.4g, Carbs: 25.7g, Fats: 38.3g

13.   Avocado Papaya Smoothie

Ingredients:

- 1 papaya, chopped
- ½ avocado, chopped
- 1 cup of plain yogurt, fat-free
- 1 tsp of coconut extract
- 1 tsp of flaxseeds, ground

Preparation:

Combine all inredients in a food processor except flaxseeds. Blend for 1 minute or until smooth. Transfer to a serving glasses and top with flaxseeds. Refigerate 30 minutes before serving.

Nutrition information per serving: Kcal: 380, Protein: 15.1g, Carbs: 68.2g, Fats: 10.7g

14.   Tuna Steaks

Ingredients:

- 4 tuna steaks, about 6 oz each
- ½ tsp of lime zest, finely grated
- 1 garlic clove, crushed
- 2 tsp olive oil
- 1 tsp of cumin, ground
- 1 tsp of coriander, ground
- ¼ tsp of black pepper, ground
- 1 tbsp lime juice

For avocado relish:

- 1 tbsp of fresh coriander, chopped
- 1 small avocado, pitted, peeled and chopped
- 1 small red onion, finely chopped

Preparation:

Trim the skin from the tuna steaks, then rinse and pat dry on absorbent kitchen paper.

In a small bowl, mix together the lime zest, garlic, olive oil, cumin, ground coriander and pepper to make a paste.

Spread the paste thinly on both sides of the tuna. Cook the tuna steaks for 5 minutes, turning once, on a foil-covered barbecue rack over hot coals, or in an oiled, ridged grill pan over high heat, in batches if necessary. Cook for another 4-5 minutes, drain on kitchen paper and transfer to a serving plate.

Sprinkle the lime juice and sprigs of fresh coriander over the cooked fish. Serve the tuna steaks with avocado relish and wedges of lime and tomato.

Avocado Relish:

To make avocado relish, peel and chop small, ripe avocado. Mix in 1 tablespoon of lime juice, 1 tablespoon of freshly chopped coriander, 1 small, finely chopped red onion and some fresh mango or tomato. Season to taste.

Nutrition information per serving: Kcal: 239, Protein: 42.3g, Carbs: 0.5g, Fats: 8.4g

15.   Vegetarian Chili Beans

Ingredients:

- 2 small fresh red chillies, finely chopped

- 1 medium-sized green bell pepper, diced

- 14 oz can red kidney beans, rinsed

- 14 oz can tomatoes, diced

- 4 oz of tomato pasta sauce

- 1 tbsp of vegetable oil

- 2 garlic cloves, crushed

Preparation:

Heat the oil in a heavy-based pan and cook the garlic, chilli and onion for 3 minutes, or until the onion is golden.

Add the remaining ingredients, bring to a boil, then reduce the heat to simmer for 15 minutes, or until thickened.

Nutrition information per serving: Kcal: 190, Protein: 9.4g, Carbs: 34.5g, Fats: 1.6g

16.   Vegetable Strudel

Ingredients:

- 1 large eggplant

- 1 medium-sized red bell pepper, chopped

- 3 zucchini, sliced lengthwise

- 2 tbsps olive oil

- 6 sheets filo pastry

- 1¾ oz baby English spinach leaves

- 2 oz of feta cheese, sliced

Preparation:

Slice the eggplant lengthwise. Sprinkle with salt and leave for 20 minutes (to draw out the bitterness). Rinse well and pat dry.

Cut the pepper into large flat pieces and place, skin side up, under a hot grill until the skin blackens and blisters. Put in a plastic bag, then peel the skin away. Brush the eggplant and zucchini slices with some of the olive oil and grill for 5-10 minutes, or until golden brown. Set aside to cool. Preheat the oven to moderately hot, about 375°F.

Brush one sheet of filo pastry at a time with olive oil, then lay them on top of each other. Place half the eggplant slices lengthwise down the center of the filo and top with layers of zucchini, pepper, spinach, and feta cheese. Repeat the layers until the vegetable and cheese are used up. Tuck in the ends of the pastry, then roll up like a parcel. Brush lightly with oil, place on a baking tray and bake for 35 minutes, or until golden brown.

Nutrition information per serving: Kcal: 287, Protein: 16.3g, Carbs: 38.2g, Fats: 2.8g

17.   Stuffed Field Mushrooms

Ingredients:

- 4 large field mushrooms

- 1 oz of butter

- 1 leek, sliced

- 3 garlic cloves, crushed

- 2 tsp of cumin seeds

- 1 tsp fresh coriander, ground

- ¼ tsp of chilli powder

- 2 medium-sized tomatoes, chopped

- 2 cups of mixed vegetables, frozen

- ½ cup of white rice, pre-cooked

- 1 oz of Cheddar cheese, grated

- ¼ cup Parmesan cheese, grated

- ¼ cup of cashews, chopped

Preparation:

Preheat the oven to 400°F. Wipe the mushrooms with a paper towel. Remove the stalks and chop them finely.

Melt the butter in a pan. Add the chopped mushroom stalks and leek and cook for 2-3 minutes, or until soft. Mix in the garlic, cumin seeds, ground coriander and chili powder and cook for 1 minute, or until the mixture is fragrant.

Stir in the tomato and frozen vegetables. Bring to a boil, reduce the heat and simmer for 5 minutes. Stir in the rice and season well.

Spoon the mixture into the mushroom caps, sprinkle with the Cheddar and Parmesan and bake for 15 minutes, or until the cheese has melted. Scatter with the cashews and serve.

Nutrition information per serving: Kcal: 180, Protein: 3.4g, Carbs: 6.6g, Fats: 3.7g

18.   Chickpea Burgers

Ingredients:

- 14 oz chickpeas, soaked
- 1 cup of red lentils
- 1 tbsp of vegetable oil
- 2 onions, sliced
- 1 tsp cumin, ground
- 1 tsp of garam masala
- 1 large egg
- ¼ cup of fresh parsley, chopped
- 2 tbsp fresh coriander, ground
- 6 oz of stale breadcrumbs
- Plain flour, for dusting

Preparation:

Add the lentils to a large pan of boiling water and simmer for 8 minutes, or until tender. Drain well. Heat the oil in a pan and cook the onion for 3 minutes, or until soft. Add the ground spices and stir until fragrant. Cool the mixture slightly.

Place the chickpeas, egg, onion mixture and half the lentils in a food processor. Process for 20 seconds, or until smooth. Transfer to a bowl. Stir in the remaining lentils, parsley, coriander and breadcrumbs. Mix well. Divide into 10 portions.

Shape the portions into round patties. (If the mixture is too soft, chill for 15 minutes, or until firm.) Toss the patties in flour, shaking off the excess. Place on a lightly greased hot barbecue grill or hotplate. Cook for 3-4 minutes on each side, or until browned.

Nutrition information per serving: Kcal: 127, Protein: 5.4g, Carbs: 24.6g, Fats: 1.3g

19.   Moroccan Couscous

Ingredients:

- 2 tbsp olive oil

- 2 cloves garlic, crushed

- 1 small red chilli, diced

- 1 leek, thinly sliced

- 2 small fennel bulbs, sliced

- 2 tsp ground cumin

- 1 tsp ground coriander

- 1 tsp ground turmeric

- 1 tspgaram masala

- 11 oz sweet potato, chopped

- 2 parsnips, sliced

- 1½ cups vegetable stock

- 2 zucchini, thickly sliced

- 8 oz broccoli, cut into florets

- 2 tomatoes, peeled and chopped

- 1 red pepper, chopped

- 14 oz can chickpeas, drained

- 2 tbsp chopped fresh flat-leaf parsley

- 2 tbsp chopped fresh lemon thyme

Couscous:

- 1¼ cups instant couscous

- 1 oz butter

- 1 cup hot vegetable stock

Preparation:

Heat the oil in a large pan and add the garlic, chilli, leek and fennel. Cook over medium heat for 10 minutes, or until the leek and fennel are soft and golden brown.

Add the cumin, coriander, turmeric, garam masala, sweet potato and parsnip. Cook for 5 minutes, stirring to coat the vegetables with spices.

Add the vegetable stock and simmer, covered, for 15 minutes. Stir in the zucchini, broccoli, tomato, pepper and chickpeas. Simmer, uncovered, for 30 minutes, or until the vegetables are tender. Stir in the herbs.

Put the couscous and butter in a bowl. Pour in the stock and leave to absorb for 5 minutes. Fluff gently with a fork to separate the grains. Make the couscous into a 'nest' on each plate and serve the spicy vegetables in the middle.

Nutrition information per serving: Kcal: 219, Protein: 6.5g, Carbs: 40g, Fats: 3g

20.   Nut Roast

Ingredients:

- 2 tbsp olive oil

- 1 large onion, diced

- 2 cloves garlic, crushed

- 10 oz field mushrooms, finely chopped

- 6½ oz raw cashews

- 6½ ozbrazil nuts

- 1 cup grated Cheddar

- ¼ cup freshly grated Parmesan

- 1 egg, lightly beaten

- 2 tbsp chopped fresh chives

- 1 cup fresh wholemeal breadcrumbs

Tomato Sauce:

- 1 floz olive oil

- 1 onion, finely chopped

- 1 clove garlic, crushed

- 13 fire roasted tomatoes, chopped

- 1 tbsp tomato paste

- 1 tsp caster sugar

Preparation:

Grease a 5½ x 8½ inches loaf tin and line the base with baking paper. Heat the oil in a frying pan and add the onion, garlic and mushrooms. Fry until soft, then allow to cool.

Process the nuts in a food processor until finely chopped, but do not overprocess. Preheat the oven to moderate 350 degrees.

Mix together the nuts, mushroom mixture, cheese, egg, chives and breadcrumbs. Press firmly into the loaf tin and bake for 15 minutes, or until firm. Leave in the tin for 5 minutes, then turn out.

To make the sauce, heat the oil in a pan and add the onion and garlic. Fry for 5 minutes, or until soft but not brown. Add the chopped tomatoes, tomato paste, sugar and 1/3 cup of water. Simmer for 3-5 minutes, or until the sauce has slightly thickened. Season to taste with salt and pepper. Serve the tomato sauce with the sliced nut roast.

Nutrition information per serving: Kcal: 297, Protein: 12g, Carbs: 24g, Fats: 14g

21.   Tomato Salsa Chickpeas

Ingredients:

- 2 cups chickpeas

- 1 small onion, chopped

- 2 cloves garlic, crushed

- 2 tbsp chopped fresh parsley

- 1 tbsp chopped fresh coriander

- 2 tsp ground cumin

- ½ tsp baking powder

- Oil, for deep-frying

Hummus:

- 14 oz chickpeas

- 2-3 tbsp lemon juice

- 2 tbsp olive oil

- 2 cloves garlic, crushed

- 3 tbsp tahini

Tomato salsa:

- 2 tomatoes, peeled and finely chopped

- ¼ cucumber, finely chopped

- ½ green pepper, finely chopped

- 2 tbsp chopped fresh parsley

- 1 tsp sugar

- 2 tspchilli sauce

- Grated rind and juice of 1 lemon

Preparation:

Soak the chickpeas in 3 cups of water for at least 4 hours. Drain and mix in a food processor for 30 seconds, or until finely ground.

Add the onion, garlic, parsley, coriander, cumin, baking powder and 1 tbsp water, and process for 10 seconds, or until the mixture forms a rough paste. Cover and set aside for 30 minutes.

To make the hummus, place the drained chickpeas, lemon juice, oil and garlic in a food processor. Season and process for 20-30 seconds, or until smooth. Add the tahini and process for a further 10 seconds.

To make the tomato salsa, mix together all the ingredients and season with plenty of freshly ground black pepper.

Shape heaped tablespoons of the falafel mixture into balls. Squeeze out the excess moisture. Heat the oil in a deep, heavy-based pan, until a cube of bread browns in 15 seconds. Lower the falafel into the oil in batches of five. Cook for 3-4 minutes each batch. When well-browned, remove with a large slotted spoon. Drain on paper towels and serve hot or cold with Lebanese bread, hummus and tomato salsa.

Nutrition information per serving: Kcal: 150, Protein: 3.9g, Carbs: 15.2g, Fats: 6g

22.   Steamed Potato Frittata

Ingredients:

- 1 tbsp olive oil

- 2 cloves garlic, crushed

- 1 small red onion, chopped

- 1 small red pepper, chopped

- 1 lb roasted, boiled or steamed potatoes, thickly sliced

- ¼ cup chopped fresh parsley

- 6 eggs, lightly beaten

- ¼ cup grated Parmesan

Preparation:

Heat the oil in a large, heavy-based, non-stick frying pan. Add the garlic, onion and pepper and stir over medium heat for 2-3 minutes. Add the potato slices and cook for 2-3 minutes more. Stir in the parsley and spread the mixture evenly in the pan.

Beat the eggs with 2 tbsp water, pour into the pan and cook over medium heat for 15 minutes, without burning the base.

Preheat the grill to high. Sprinkle the Parmesan over the frittata and grill for a few minutes to cook the egg and lightly brown. Cut into wedges to serve.

Nutrition information per serving: Kcal: 208, Protein: 11g, Carbs: 17g, Fats: 10g

23.   Cannellini Beans Sausages

Ingredients:

- 1 tbsp sunflower oil

- 1 small onion, finely chopped

- 1¾ oz mushrooms, finely chopped

- ½ red pepper, deseeded and finely chopped

- 14 oz cannellini beans, rinsed and drained

- 3½ oz fresh breadcrumbs

- 3½ oz Cheddar cheese, grated

- 1 tsp dried mixed herbs

- 1 egg yolk

- All-purpose flour, to coat

- Oil, for cooking

Preparation:

Heat the oil in a pan and cooked the prepared onion, mushrooms and red pepper until softened.

Mash the cannellini beans in a large mixing bowl. Add the chopped onion, mushroom and red pepper mixture, and the breadcrumbs, cheese, herbs and egg yolk, and mix together well.

Press the mixture together with your fingers and shape into eight sausages.

Roll each sausage in the seasoned flour. Chill for at least 30 minutes.

Barbecue the sausages on a sheet of oiled foil set over medium-hot coals for 15-20 minutes, turning and basting frequently with oil, until golden.

Split the bread rolls down the middle and insert a layer of fried onions. Place the sausages in the rolls and serve.

Nutrition information per serving: Kcal: 213, Protein: 8g, Carbs: 19g, Fats: 12g

24.   Grated Pupkin Frittata

Ingredients:

- 3 tbsp olive oil
- 1 onion, finely chopped
- 1 small carrot, grated
- 1 small zucchini, grated
- 1 cup grated pumpkin
- 1/3 cup finely-diced Cheddar cheese
- 5 eggs, lightly beaten

Preparation:

Heat 2 tablespoons of the oil in a pan and cook the onion for 5 minutes, or until soft. Add the carrot, zucchini and pumpkin and cook over low heat, covered, for 3 minutes. Transfer to a bowl and allow to cool. Stir in the cheese and plenty of salt and pepper. Add the eggs.

Heat the remaining oil in a small non-stick frying pan. Add the frittata mixture and shake the pan to spread it evenly. Reduce to low and cook for 15-20 minutes, or until set almost all the way through. Tilt the pan and lift the edges occasionally   to   allow   the   uncooked   egg   to   flow underneath. Brown the top under a preheated hot grill. Cut into wedges and serve immediately.

Nutrition information per serving: Kcal: 114, Protein: 10g, Carbs: 6g, Fats: 5g

25.   Colorful Kebabs

Ingredients:

- 1 red pepper, deseeded

- 1 yellow pepper, deseeded

- 1 green pepper, deseeded

- 1 small onion

- 8 cherry tomatoes

- 3½ oz wild mushrooms

Seasoned oil:

- 6 tbsp olive oil

- 1 garlic clove, crushed

- ½ tsp mixed dried herbs

Preparation:

Cut the red, yellow and green peppers into 1-inch pieces.

Peel the onion and cut into wedges, leaving the root end just intact to help keep the wedges together.

Thread the pepper pieces, onion wedges, tomatoes and mushrooms onto skewers, alternating the colors of the peppers.

To make the seasoned oil, mix together the olive oil, garlic and mixed herbs in a small bowl. Brush the mixture liberally over the kebabs.

Barbecue the kebabs over medium-hot coals for 10-15 minutes, brushing with the seasoned oil and turning the skewers frequently.

Transfer the vegetable kebabs onto warmed serving plates.

Nutrition information per serving: Kcal: 257, Protein: 3g, Carbs: 26g, Fats: 16g

26.   Garlic Potato Wedges

Ingredients:

- 3 large baking potatoes, scrubbed
- 4 tbsp olive oil
- 2 tbsp butter
- 2 garlic cloves, chopped
- 1 tbsp chopped fresh rosemary
- 1 tbsp chopped fresh parsley
- 1 tbsp chopped fresh thyme
- Salt and pepper

Preparation:

Bring a large saucepan of water to a boil, add the potatoes and parboil them for 10 minutes. Drain the potatoes, refresh under cold water and then drain them again thoroughly.

Transfer the potatoes to a chopping board. When cold enough to handle, cut into thick wedges, but do not peel.

Heat the oil, butter and garlic in a small saucepan. Cook gently until the garlic begins to brown, then remove the pan from the heat.

Stir the herbs, and salt and pepper to taste, into the mixture in the saucepan.

Brush the warm garlic and herb mixture generously over the parboiled potato wedges.

Barbecue the potatoes over hot coals for 10-15 minutes, brushing liberally with any of the remaining garlic and herb mixture, or until the potato wedges are just tender.

Transfer the garlic potato wedges to a warm serving plate and serve as a starter or side dish.

Nutrition information per serving: Kcal: 336, Protein: 3.9g, Carbs: 32.4g, Fats: 26.8g

27.   Saffron Risotto

Ingredients:

- Large pinch of good-quality saffron threads

- 16 floz boiling water

- 1 tsp salt

- 2 tbsp butter

- 2 tbsp olive oil

- 1 large onion, very finely chopped

- 3 tbsp pine kernels

- 12 oz long grain rice

- 2oz sultanas

- 6 green cardamom pods, shells lightly cracked

- 6 cloves

- Pepper

- Very finely chopped fresh coriander or flat-leaved parsley, to garnish

Preparation:

Toast the saffron threads in a dry frying pan over a medium heat, stirring, for 2 minutes, until they give off an aroma.

Immediately tip out onto a plate.

Pour the boiling water into a measuring jug, stir in the saffron and salt and leave to infuse for 30 minutes.

Melt the butter and oil in a frying pan over a medium-high heat. Add the onion. Cook for about 5 minutes, stirring.

Lower the heat, stir the pine kernels into the onions and continue cooking for 2 minutes, stirring, until the nuts just begin to turn a golden color. Take care not to burn them.

Stir in the rice, coating all the grains with oil. Stir for 1 minute, then add the sultanas, cardamom pods and cloves. Pour in the saffron-flavored water and bring to a boil. Lower the heat, cover and simmer for 15 minutes without removing the lid.

Remove from the heat. Leave to stand for 5 minutes without uncovering. Remove the lid and check that the rice is tender, the liquid has been absorbed and the surface has small indentations all over.

Fluff up the rice and adjust the seasoning. Stir in the herbs and serve.

Nutrition information per serving: Kcal: 347, Protein: 5g, Carbs: 60g, Fats: 11g

28.   Ginger Charred Chicken

Ingredients:

- 4 chicken breasts, skinned and boned

- 2 tbsp curry paste

- 1 tbsp sunflower oil, plus extra for cooking

- 1 tbsp brown sugar

- 1 tsp ground ginger

- ½ tsp ground cumin

Yogurt Topping:

- ¼ cucumber

- Salt

- ½ cup of low-fat natural yogurt

- ¼ tsp chilli powder

Preparation:

Place the chicken breasts between two sheets of baking paper or clingfilm. Pound them with the flat side of a meat mallet or rolling pin to flatten them. Mix together the curry paste, oil, brown sugar, ginger and cumin in a small bowl.

Spread the mixture over both sides of the chicken and then set aside until required.

To make the yogurt topping, peel the cucumber and scoop out the seeds with a spoon. Grate the cucumber flesh, sprinkle with salt, place in a sieve and leave to stand for 10 minutes. Rinse off the salt and squeeze out any remaining moisture by pressing the cucumber with the base of a glass or the back of a spoon. In a small bowl, mix the grated cucumber with the natural yogurt and stir in the chilli powder. Leave to chill until needed.

Transfer the chicken pieces to an oiled rack and barbecue over hot coals for 10 minutes, turning once.

Serve the chicken with yogurt topping.

Nutrition information per serving: Kcal: 228, Protein: 28g, Carbs: 12g, Fats: 8g

29.   Apples Stuffed with Nuts and Cherries

Ingredients:

- 4 medium cooking apples

- 2 tbsp chopped walnuts

- 2 tbsp ground almonds

- 2 tbsp light muscovado sugar

- 2 tbsp chopped cherries

- 2 tbsp chopped crystallized ginger

- 4 tbsp butter

- Single cream or thick natural yogurt, to serve

Preparation:

Core the apples and, using a sharp knife, score each one around the middle to prevent the apple skins from splitting during barbecuing.

To make the filling, in a small bowl, mix together the walnuts, almonds, sugar, cherries and ginger.

Spoon the filling mixture into each apple, pushing it down into the hollowed-out core. Mound a little of the filling mixture on top of each apple.

Place each apple on a large square of double-thickness foil and generously dot with the butter. Wrap up the foil so that each apple is completely enclosed.

Barbecue the parcels containing the apples over hot coals for about 25-30 minutes, or until tender.

Transfer the apples to warm individual serving plates. Serve with lashings of whipped single cream or thick natural yogurt.

Nutrition information per serving: Kcal: 294, Protein: 3g, Carbs: 31g, Fats: 18g

30.   Creamy Banana Dessert

Ingredients:

- 4 bananas

- 2 passion fruit

- 4 tbsp orange juice

- 4 tbsp orange-flavored liqueur

- Creamy topping:

- 5 floz double cream

- 3 tbsp icing sugar

- 2 tbsp orange-flavored liqueur

Preparation:

To make the orange-flavored cream, pour the double cream into a mixing bowl and sprinkle over the icing sugar. Whisk the mixture until it is standing in soft peaks. Carefully fold in the orange-flavored liqueur and chill in the refrigerator until needed.

Peel the bananas and place each one onto a sheet of foil.

Cut the passion fruit in half and squeeze the juice of each half over each banana. Spoon over the orange juice and liqueur. Fold the foil carefully over the top of the bananas so that they are completely enclosed.

Place the parcels on a baking tray and cook over hot coals for 10-15 minutes, or until they are just tender (test by inserting a cocktail stick or a toothpick). Transfer the foil parcels to warm, individual serving plates. Open out the foil parcels and then serve immediately with the orange-flavored cream.

Nutrition information per serving: Kcal: 380, Protein: 2g, Carbs: 43g, Fats: 19g

31.   Thick Red Lentil Soup

Ingredients:

- 2 tbsp butter

- 2 garlic cloves, crushed

- 1 onion, chopped

- ½ tsp turmeric

- 1 tsp garam masala

- ¼ tsp chili powder

- 1 tsp ground cumin

- 2 lb of chopped tomatoes

- 7 oz red lentils

- 2 tsp lemon juice

- 1 pint vegetable stock

- 10 floz coconut milk

- Salt and pepper

For serving:

- Fresh chopped coriander

- Lemon slices

Preparation:

Melt the butter in a large saucepan. Add the garlic and onion and sauté, stirring, for 2-3 minutes. Add the turmeric, garam masala, chili powder and cumin and cook for another 30 seconds.

Chop the tomatoes and stir into the pan with the red lentils, lemon juice, vegetable stock and coconut stock and bring to a boil.

Reduce the heat to low and simmer the soup, uncovered for about 25-30 minutes until the lentils are tender and cooked.

Season to taste with salt and pepper and ladle the soup into warm serving bowls. Garnish with chopped coriander and lemon slices and serve immediately with warm naan bread.

Nutrition information per serving: Kcal: 284, Protein: 16g, Carbs: 38g, Fats: 9g

32. Chicken Soup

Ingredients:

- 12oz minced chicken
- 1 tbsp tomato sauce
- 1 tsp grated fresh root ginger
- 1 garlic clove, finely chopped
- 2 tsp sherry
- 2 spring onions, chopped
- 1 tsp sesame oil
- 1 egg white
- ½ tsp rice flour
- ½ tsp sugar
- 35 wonton skins
- 2½ pints chicken stock
- 1 spring onion, shredded
- 1 small carrot, thinly sliced

Preparation:

Put the chicken, ginger, garlic, sherry, spring onions, sesame oil, egg white, rice flour and sugar in a bowl and mix well. Place a small spoonful of the filling in the center of each wonton skin. Dampen the edges. Gather up each one to form a pouch to enclose the filling.

Cook the wontons in boiling water for 1 minute or until they float to the surface. Remove with a slotted spoon.

Pour the chicken stock into a saucepan and bring to a boil. Add the spring onion, carrot and wontons to the soup. Simmer gently for 2 minutes, then serve.

Nutrition information per serving: Kcal: 101, Protein: 14g, Carbs: 3g, Fats: 4g

33.   Tomato Kebabs

Ingredients:

- 1 lb rump or sirloin steak

- 16 cherry tomatoes

- 16 large green olives, stoned

- Salt and freshly ground black pepper

- Focaccia bread, to serve

- 4 tbsp olive oil

- 1 tbsp sherry vinegar

- 1 garlic clove, crushed

- 1 tbsp olive oil

- 1 tbsp sherry vinegar

- 1 garlic clove, crushed

- 6 plum tomatoes, skinned, deseeded anc chopped

- 2 green olives, stoned and sliced

- 1 tbsp chopped fresh parsley

- 1 tbsp lemon juice

Preparation:

Trim any fat from the meat and cut into about 24 even-sized pieces. Thread the meat into 8 skewers, alternating it with cherry tomatoes and the stoned whole olives.

To make the paste, in a bowl combine the oil, vinegar, garlic, and salt and pepper to taste.

To make the fresh tomato relish, heat the oil in a small saucepan and cook the onion and garlic for 3-4 minutes until softened. Add the tomatoes and sliced olives and cook for 2-3 minutes until the tomatoes are softened slightly. Stir in the parsley and lemon juice, and season with salt and pepper to taste. Set aside and keep warm or leave to chill.

Barbecue the skewers on an oiled rack over hot coals for 5-10 minutes, basting and turning frequently. Serve with the tomato relish and slices of focaccia.

Nutrition information per serving: Kcal: 166, Protein: 12g, Carbs: 1g, Fats: 12g

34.   Pork with Rice

Ingredients:

- 14oz lean pork fillet

- 3 tbsp orange marmalade

- Grated zest and juice of 1 orange

- 1 tbsp white wine vinegar

- 1 tsp of Tabasco sauce

- Salt and pepper

- 1 tbsp olive oil

- 1 small onion, chopped

- 1 small, green pepper, deseeded and thinly sliced

- 1 tbspcornflour

- 5 floz orange juice

Serving:

- Cooked rice

- Mixed salad leaves

Preparation:

Place a large piece of double thickness foil in a shallow dish.

Put the pork fillet in the center of the foil and season to taste. Heat the marmalade, orange zest and juice, vinegar and Tabasco sauce in a small pan, stirring, until the marmalade melts and the ingredients combine. Pour the mixture over the pork and wrap the meat in the foil. Seal the parcel well so that the juices cannot run out. Place over hot coals and barbecue for 25 minutes, turning the parcel occasionally.

For the sauce, heat the oil in a pan and cook the onion for 2-3 minutes. Add the pepper and cook for 3-4 minutes. Remove the pork from the foil and place on the racke. Pour the juices into the pan with the sauce. Continue barbecuing the pork for another 10-20 minutes, turning, until cooked through and golden.

In a bowl, mix the cornflour into a paste with a little orange juice. Add to the sauce with the remaining cooking juices. Cook, stirring, until it thickens. Slice the pork, spoon over the sauce and serve with rice and salad leaves.

Nutrition information per serving: Kcal: 230, Protein: 19g, Carbs: 16g, Fats: 9g

35. French Croissant

Ingredients:

- 2 pounds of all-purpose flour
- 1 small pack of dry yeast
- 2 tsp   salt
- 5 tbsp oil
- 1 whole egg
- 1 ½ cup of milk
- 1 cup   of water
- 1 cup butter
- 1 whole egg
- 1 egg   yolk
- 1 cup   of organic cocoa cream

Preparation:

In a small bowl combine the yeast with 1/2 cup of warm milk, 1 tsp of sugar, and 1 tsp of all-purpose flour. Allow it to stand for about 30 minutes. Combine the yeast with other ingredients and make a smooth dough. Shape 16 little bowls and roll out the dough.

Place 1 tbsp of cocoa cream at the center of each croissant and roll in.

Preheat the oven to 400 degrees and bake the croissants for about 15 minutes.

Meanwhile, combine 1 egg and 1 egg yolk in a bowl. Spread this mixture, with a kitchen brush, over each croissant before removing them from the oven.

Nutrition information per serving: Kcal: 491, Protein: 10g, Carbs: 59g, Fats: 23.5g

36. Seafood Risotto with Turmeric

Ingredients:

- 1 cup of rice

- 1 cup of fresh seafood mix

- ½ cup of peas, cooked

- 1 small tomato

- ½ bell pepper, finely chopped

- 1 tbsp of ground turmeric

- Salt to taste

Preparation:

Briefly boil the seafood mix, for about 3-4 minutes. Drain and set aside.

Add one cup of rice and 3 cups of water in a deep pot. Bring it to a boil and cook for about 10 minutes, or until half of the water has evaporated.

Meanwhile, peel and finely chop the tomato and bell pepper. Mix with peas in a bowl and season with salt.

Combine this mixture with rice, add seafood mix, one tablespoon of ground turmeric and cook until all the water has evaporated. You can serve with some grated Parmesan cheese.

Nutrition information per serving: Kcal: 198, Protein: 4.8g, Carbs: 42.7g, Fats: 0.6g

37. Lentil and Chickpea Salad with Fresh Lemon Juice

Ingredients:

- ½ cup of cooked lentils

- ½ cup of cooked chickpeas

- ½ red onion, finely chopped

- 1 cup of lettuce, finely chopped

- 3 tbsp of fresh lemon juice

- 2 tbsp of olive oil

Preparation:

First you will have to cook the lentils. For ½ cup of dry lentils, you will need 1 ½ cup of water, because the lentils will double in size. Bring it to a boil, reduce the heat and cook for about 15-20 minutes, or until the lentils have softened. Remove from the heat and drain. Allow it to cool for a while.

Place all the ingredients in a bowl and mix well. Before serving, add three tablespoons of fresh lemon juice and two tablespoons of olive oil. Toss well to coat.

Nutrition information per serving: Kcal: 246, Protein: 11.3g, Carbs: 31.5g, Fats: 8.9g

38.   Quick Homemade Polenta

Ingredients:

- 17oz corn flour

- 5 cups of water

- 5 tbsp of olive oil

- A pinch of salt

Preparation:

Bring five cups of water to a boiling point. Add salt, olive oil, and reduce the heat to medium. Slowly whisk in the corn flour. Cook until the mixture thickens, stirring often. Remove from the heat and serve.

Nutrition information per serving: Kcal: 334, Protein: 4.8g, Carbs: 52.9g, Fats: 12.7g

39.   Lean Potato Salad with Olive Oil

Ingredients:

- 2 medium-sized potatoes, boiled

- 5 spring onions, finely chopped

- 1 small red onion, peeled and sliced

- Olive oil to taste

- Salt to taste

- Pepper to taste

Preparation:

First you will have to boil the potatoes. Peel and thoroughly rinse the potatoes. Slice and transfer to a deep pot. Add just enough water to cover. Bring it to a boil and cook for about 15 minutes, or until the potatoes have softened. Remove from the heat and drain. Allow it to cool for a while.

Meanwhile, prepare the onions. Trim the roots away and strip off any extra outer leaves. Finely chop and combine with potatoes.

Peel and slice the onion. Add to the salad mixture. Season with olive oil, salt and pepper to taste. You can add a few drops of fresh lemon juice, but this is optional.

Serve cold.

Nutrition information per serving: Kcal: 259, Protein: 3.1g, Carbs: 26.3g, Fats: 17g

40.   Almond Salad

Ingredients:

- ½ pear sliced

- 1 kiwi, peeled and sliced

- Few cherry tomatoes, halved

- ½ cup of wild berries

- ½ cup of nut mix

- ½ green bell pepper, sliced

- For the dressing:

- 2 tbsp of honey

- ¼ cup of fresh lime juice

- 1 tsp of mustard

Preparation:

Whisk fresh lime juice, mustard and honey with a fork.

In a large bowl, combine the vegetables and add the dressing. Toss well to combine.

If you're not a big fan of fruit/vegetable mixture, you can easily skip the vegetables and create a beautiful fruit salad.

However, you should also replace the mustard dressing with few drops of fresh lemon juice and sugar.

Nutrition information per serving: Kcal: 135, Protein: 1.9g, Carbs: 33.4g, Fats: 0.9g

41.   Mackerel with Potatoes and Greens

Ingredients:

- 4 medium-sized mackerels, skin on

- 1 lb of fresh spinach, torn

- 5 large potatoes, peeled and sliced

- ¼ cup (divided in half) of extra virgin olive oil

- 3 garlic cloves, crushed

- 1 tsp of dried rosemary, finely chopped

- 2 springs of fresh mint leaves, chopped

- 1 lemon, juiced

- 1 tsp of sea salt

Preparation:

Peel and slice potatoes. Make the base layer in a deep, heavy-bottomed pot. Spread one-half of your olive oil over potatoes. Now add torn spinach and top with the remaining olive oil. Add crushed garlic, rosemary, mint, and lemon juice.

Generously sprinkle some salt over mackerels. Make the final layer in your pot and cover.

Cook for 45 minutes over medium-low heat.

Nutrition information per serving: Kcal: 244, Protein: 14g, Carbs: 19.2g, Fats: 12g

42. Slow Cooked White Beans

Ingredients:

- 1 lb of white peas

- 4 slices of dried beef

- 1 large onion, finely chopped

- 1 garlic clove, crushed

- 1 medium-sized red bell pepper, finely chopped

- 1 small chili pepper, finely chopped

- 2 tbsp of all-purpose flour

- 2 tbsp of butter

- 1 tbsp of cayenne pepper

- 3 bay leaves, dried

- 1 tsp of salt

- ½ tsp of freshly ground black pepper

Preparation:

Melt two tablespoons of butter in a slow cooker. Add chopped onion, crushed garlic, and stir well. Now add dried beef, peas, finely chopped red bell pepper, chili pepper, bay leaves, salt, and pepper. Gently stir in two tablespoons of flour and add three cups of water.

Securely close the lid and cook for 8-9 hours on low setting or 5 hours on high setting.

Nutrition information per serving: Kcal: 210, Protein: 4g, Carbs: 24g, Fats: 12g

43.   Collard Greens Rolls

Ingredients:

- 1.5 lb of collard greens, steamed
- 1 lb lean ground beef
- 2 small onions, peeled and finely chopped
- ½ cup long grain rice
- 2 tbsp of olive oil
- 1 tsp of salt
- ½ tsp of freshly ground black pepper
- 1 tsp of mint leaves, finely chopped

Preparation:

Boil a large pot of water and gently the greens. Briefly cook, for 2-3 minutes. Drain and gently squeeze the greens and set aside.

In a large bowl, combine the ground beef with finely chopped onions, rice, salt, pepper, and mint leaves.

Oil a deep pot with some olive oil. Place leaves on your work surface, vein side up. Use one tablespoon of the meat mixture and place it in the bottom center of each leaf. Fold the sides over and roll up tightly. Tuck in the sides and gently transfer to a pot.

Cover and cook for one hour over a medium heat.

Nutrition information per serving: Kcal: 156, Protein: 5.2g, Carbs: 21g, Fats: 7g

44.   Whole Chicken Stew

Ingredients:

- 1 whole chicken, 3 lbs

- 10 oz of fresh broccoli

- 7 oz cauliflower florets

- 1 large onion, peeled and finely chopped

- 1 large potato, peeled and chopped

- 3 medium-sized carrots, sliced

- 1 large tomato, peeled and chopped

- A handful of yellow wax beans, whole

- A handful of fresh parsley, finely chopped

- ¼ cup of extra virgin olive oil

- 2 tsp of salt

- ½ tsp of freshly ground black pepper

- 1 tbsp of cayenne pepper

Preparation:

Clean the chicken and generously sprinkle with some salt.
Set aside.

Grease the bottom of a heavy bottomed pot with three tablespoons of olive oil. Add finely chopped onion and stir-fry for 3-4 minutes and then add sliced carrot. Continue to cook for five more minutes.

Now add the remaining oil, vegetables, salt, black pepper, cayenne pepper, and top with chicken. Add one cup of water and cover.

Simmer for one hour over medium heat.

Nutrition information per serving: Kcal: 290, Protein: 31g, Carbs: 39g, Fats: 6g

45.   Veal Okra with Artichokes

Ingredients:

- 7 oz veal shoulder, blade chops

- 1 lb okra, rinsed and trimmed

- 3 large artichokes, whole

- 2 medium-sized tomatoes, halved

- 2-3 fresh cauliflower florets

- 2 cups of vegetable broth

- A handful of fresh broccoli

- 3 tablespoons of extra virgin olive oil

- 1 tsp of Himalayan salt

- ½ tsp of freshly ground black pepper

Preparation:

Grease a deep pot with three tablespoons of olive oil. Set aside.

Cut each okra pod in half lengthwise and place in a pot. Add tomato halves, artichokes, cauliflower florets, a handful of fresh broccoli, and top with meat chops.

Season with salt and pepper and add two cups of vegetable broth. Give it a good stir and cover.

Cook for 45 minutes over medium-high heat, or two hours over low temperature.

Nutrition information per serving: Kcal: 281, Protein: 19.6g, Carbs: 17.4g, Fats: 15.5g

ADDITIONAL TITLES FROM THIS AUTHOR

70 Effective Meal Recipes to Prevent and Solve Being Overweight: Burn Fat Fast by Using Proper Dieting and Smart Nutrition

By

Joe Correa CSN

48 Acne Solving Meal Recipes: The Fast and Natural Path to Fixing Your Acne Problems in Less Than 10 Days!

By

Joe Correa CSN

41 Alzheimer's Preventing Meal Recipes: Reduce or Eliminate Your Alzheimer's Condition in 30 Days or Less!

By

Joe Correa CSN

70 Effective Breast Cancer Meal Recipes: Prevent and Fight Breast Cancer with Smart Nutrition and Powerful Foods

By

Joe Correa CSN

www.ingramcontent.com/pod-product-compliance
Lightning Source LLC
Chambersburg PA
CBHW030246030426
42336CB00009B/275